LEXI MEYEROWITZ

Spirit Birth

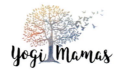

First published by Yogi Mamas in 2018

Copyright © Lexi Meyerowitz, 2018

All rights reserved. No part of this publication may be reproduced, stored or transmitted in any form or by any means, electronic, mechanical, photocopying, recording, scanning, or otherwise without written permission from the publisher. It is illegal to copy this book, post it to a website, or distribute it by any other means without permission.

Designations used by companies to distinguish their products are often claimed as trademarks. All brand names and product names used in this book and on its cover are trade names, service marks, trademarks and registered trademarks of their respective owners. The publishers and the book are not associated with any product or vendor mentioned in this book. None of the companies referenced within the book have endorsed the book.

The information provided in this book is designed to provide helpful information on the subjects discussed. This book is not meant to be used, nor should it be used, to diagnose or treat any medical condition. For diagnosis or treatment of any medical problem, consult your own physician. The publisher and author are not responsible for any specific health or allergy needs that may require medical supervision and are not liable for any damages or negative consequences from any treatment, action, application or preparation, to any person reading or following the information in this book. References are provided for informational purposes only and do not constitute endorsement of any websites or other sources. Readers should be aware that the websites listed in this book may change.

First edition

This book was professionally typeset on Reedsy.
Find out more at reedsy.com

Contents

I   The Yoga of Birth

Acknowledgements	3
Introduction	4
Manifesting Spirit	7
The 8 Limbs of Yoga for Pregnancy, Birth, and Motherhood	10
Oneness, Samadhi	17

II   Spiritual Bootcamp- Body, Mind, Spirit

15 Minute Yoga Asana Practices for the Body	21
5 Minute Yoga Practices	43
Pranayama Practices for the Breath	57
Mantras and Ideas for the Mind	60
Foods for Your Body and Baby	69

III   Spirit Initiation

Stages of Receiving Spirit, the Hero's Journey	75
Stages of Labor	80
Re-Birth in Postpartum	83

IV Final Notes

Conclusion   89
About Lexi Meyerowitz   91
Resources   95

PART I

The Yoga of Birth

Your body is where Spirit and Matter come together.

One

Acknowledgements

~~~~~

This book is dedicated to *my* Mom.

I'd like to thank my children for being my gurus, my husband for his support and edits, my friends for their love and encouragement, my students for their enthusiasm, and my mentors for their wisdom. In particular I'd like to thank: Sophia, Hana, Adam, Valentine, Masha, Andi, Shelley R., Paisley, Sujantra, Gerry, and Lisa. I'd also like to give a special thanks to my Dad for giving me invaluable strategies for completing this undertaking, and my brother for always believing in me.

Thank You, to the Universe for guiding me.

Two

Introduction

I have come to know that pregnancy is *"Spiritual Bootcamp"*. Have you also? You've most likely already had 3 or 4 trials in faith and self-love by the time you've come to this book. I believe there's a purpose to all this angst. You are going through *Spiritual Bootcamp*. What takes some people a lifetime to learn, you will be experiencing in just 9 months. Sure, you may need to have these lessons again at other times in your life, but if you can consciously do this Spiritual Workout, you'll feel stronger and more graceful in the moment and in the future.

Feeling strong and graceful as you go from "individual" to "mother", you'll carry this wisdom into your relationship with your child. You will learn about balancing opposites like boundaries and togetherness. You'll recover your values and self-worth. You'll learn about what faith means to you. Staying present and looking ahead at the same time, you'll begin to understand time differently. Sometimes you are going to learn how to ask for help and others how to say no. You'll learn how to be brave, to lean in to discomfort, and that you are part of something much bigger than yourself.

Prenatal Yoga is a boat that can help get you there safely. You are crossing the wild "river beneath the river" (*Women Who Run With the Wolves*, Estes), and you will come to the other side feeling refreshed

Introduction

and renewed. Yoga reminds us that we are spiritual beings living in physical form. Our spirit is called *Atman* or sometimes *Purusa* and it helps us tune into ourselves, the world around us, and our children. This inner wisdom shapes who we are, how we engage with the world, and what brings meaning to our lives. It prepares a woman for birth and motherhood.

For most women, birth is the great unknown. Even people who know a lot about birth see it as the unknown. I have seen OBGYNs in my Prenatal Yoga classes in San Diego and they still have trepidation about their own birth. Because, each birth is so unique it is hard to grapple with preparing for it. And so much of birth is hard to describe with words, no guide can tell us exactly what it feels like. Ultimately, when a woman prepares for birth, she is preparing for the unknown.

How does one prepare for the unknown? That is what Yoga and the journey of the hero helps us do. Most of us try to control the unknown. I know I surely did. I had all the apps, read all the books, wrote my birth plan, etc. etc. etc. But like most women, I quickly realized that I had very little control over these grand forces beyond myself.

So what then? If you don't have control, what's the point of reading this book? Is it all over- must you just accept what there is and take no action to support yourself and your baby? In Taoism, the answer is referred to as *Wei Wu Wei,* m*e*aning action without action. All movement must come from an inner stillness. When we are still, we are not reaching out of ourselves for something more, we are satisfied. We make choices without being attached to the outcome. That is where the physical, mental, and spiritual practices of Yoga help a woman uncover acceptance and illuminate her readiness to enter into the unknown. In Yoga this is called *aparigraha,* non-attachment, and it is a crucial part of your heroic journey.

Attachment will show up in different ways for each woman in pregnancy. Here's how it showed up one time during the birth of my second child. By this time I had already experienced an unmedicated, beautiful birth with my first, and I was a happy Prenatal Yoga teacher.

But, I was attached to my identity as "prenatal yoga teacher". I had a lot of expectations about what my birth "should" look like. Well, my spiritual journey doesn't do "shoulds". When my water broke and contractions wouldn't start, I needed Pitocin to get things going. I was bummed, I felt deeply saddened by this turn of events and I couldn't let go. But when I decided I had to let go of that attachment to the "shoulds" of birth, I was able to fully become present with my body. I stopped judging myself and let myself be. I silenced my inner critic, changed my language to support, and found strength and serenity. To my surprise, I was able to work with the Pitocin contractions, letting them get stronger and stronger without much more medication. With this spiritual high, I was able to ride the wave into an empowering birth experience.

Whatever your birth preferences are, and how your unique birth will unfold, this book can support you. Strength, compassion, and connection with the infinite-self are central themes to both Yoga and Birth no matter what your life and birth experiences are.

The many subtle layers the pregnant woman will traverse as she journeys closer and closer to birth will prepare her for birth itself, and for motherhood after. In this book we will look at a number of themes, including: Perspectives on Time, Discomfort, Support, Peace and Calm, Language, Mothering the Mother, the Emotional Body, Mirroring, Rhythm, Ritual, Relaxation, Spaciousness, Balance, Focus, Acceptance, and Strength.

Just as any hero has her challenges, so too does the mother. She is not alone, she is supported and held, not just by the people around her, but by something greater than herself. I hope this book will serve as a reminder and tool for you to use in your *Spiritual Bootcamp* and birth journey.

OM Shanti, Many Blessings On Your Birth,
Lexi Meyer

Three

Manifesting Spirit

In your body, the space of your womb holds spirit and matter as they dance into one. Before your child grew into your womb, your child's spirit was without form. Only in you can this child's spirit come into his/her form. This form that is created in you will grow and change as your baby evolves through the stages of life.

This sacred creation requires your body to be the bridge between the physical and non-physical worlds. As such, pregnancy can be overwhelming emotionally and spiritually as well as physically. Without the proper language to discuss this inner journey, women can feel isolated and even crazy at times. This book aims to open up the dialogue about this sacred work so that women can move past the boundaries of what is expected of them and find peace with who they are.

In some circles this work is already underway. Many women talk about feelings of connection to their children before they are born. Some even have dreams or visions. Some have a feeling that they knew they were pregnant long before they took the first test. Many of these experiences are Spirit Signals.

Spirit Signals

You may receive Spirit Signals throughout your pregnancy and birth. This is an opportunity to get to know your own way of communicating with the universe. Explore the signals, see what feels safe for you. For example, maybe there is an animal that keeps reappearing throughout your pregnancy. Once you start to become aware of this way of spirit signaling you, there will be opportunities for you to practice leaning in to it.

Spirit Signaled me when I was visiting the hospital, deciding if that's where I wanted to deliver my first daughter. I asked the Universe to please help me know. I walked out of the elevator onto the labor and delivery floor. A beautiful view greeted me through large windows. I walked closer and noticed a Hawk's nest on the ledge of the window, with a mother hawk nuzzling her babies. My heart became so warm that my body began to tingle and I felt light. This was a Spirit Signal.

If this is something that you're interested in exploring, start by asking the Universe for help. Then pay attention over the next few weeks, see any themes that keep coming up (mine was birds). These repetitive themes are probably Spirit Signals. Become aware of how you feel and notice how your response to the Spirit Signal makes you feel, better or worse. Of course, this goes without saying that if you are signaled to do something dangerous, self-defeating, or painful to someone else, this is NOT spirit and, of course, please find someone to talk to about those feelings.

***

Your body is simultaneously the home of your spirit and your baby's spirit, opening you up to a larger amount of spiritual connection than you may have had before. For some, this can be overwhelming, and it is helpful to find someone you can talk with about your experiences.

The physical movements of Yoga Asanas in this book and in a Prenatal Yoga class will help you move through these experiences, so that you don't become stuck. The breathwork and mantra meditation also helps create space for this spiritual work to flow. You're doing a great job already, and if you would like to dive deeper, this book will guide you.

Four

The 8 Limbs of Yoga for Pregnancy, Birth, and Motherhood

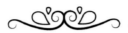

"[I am a conscious parent when I] believe that my child is here to teach me as much about myself and how I need to grow, as I am here to teach them" - Shefali Tsabary, The Conscious Parent

Most people in the West know of Yoga as physical postures we see on TV and on Billboards. Some of us know about the conscious breathing. Very few know that Yoga is actually a time-tested system to support a mindful connection between the individual self, and Truth (the consciousness of the universe).

You can paraphrase this as "Yoga means Union". There are 8 steps that lead to this union, the final step called *Samadhi*. We will go through each step, and relate each step to the process of manifesting a spirit into a human body, all of the work and wisdom that comes with this process.

Yamas- Self-Regulating Behaviors
Niyamas- Personal Observances
Asana- Yoga Postures, What Many Often Call Yoga
Pranayama- Breath Regulation

Pratyahara- Withdrawal of the Senses, Inner Awareness
Dharana- Focused Concentration
Dhyana- Meditative Absorption
Samadhi- Experiencing Oneness

The first two steps are usually worked together, and will continue to come up as you work through the rest of the book. Every woman goes through this, but women rarely talk about it. Be kind to yourself as you go through the process and recognize when some work is beyond the scope of this book. For deeper work into self-healing, self-awareness, and healthy behaviors for you, please contact a professional you trust. For some with a lot of healing work to do, it may be advised not to do this work during pregnancy. If this is the case, just skip this section and go straight to Spiritual Bootcamp.

Yamas and Niyamas- Principles of Being

The Yamas and Niyamas are the Principles of Being that we learn from the Yogic Tradition. These principles address our outer world, like how we interact with people and things in the world. These principles also address our inner world, how to focus and bring peace to our inner experience.

Explore how the Yamas and Niyamas interact in your life. Do you have violent thoughts or jealousy? Are you truthful with yourself and others? What does intimicy look like in your life- could you bring more awareness to it? The hardest one I see in my Yoga classes is *Aparigraha-* non-attachment. As the saying goes, it's the journey, not the destination. But as expecting mothers, it's hard to let go of the inner drive to have a healthy baby. Even still, we can only do so much, and the rest is out of our hands.

This is where surrender to a higher power can help (*Ishvara Pranidhana*), as well as contentment (*santosha*); this allows us to find joy in ourselves and with a higher power, rather than seeking joy outside of ourselves. Purity, self-study, and self-discipline are ways to deepen and maintain that relationship with ourselves and the higher power.

As you consider these Yamas and Niyamas, of how to be in relationship with the world and do the inner work, you may find that you need to go deeper. This book is a jumping off point to uncover how to use pregnancy as a time to let go, adapt, and embrace what is. If this is too much energy movement for you at this moment in your life, that's okay, focus on what you need to, and come back to this when you're ready- even if it's in 15 years. It can also be helpful to do this work with a trained professional like an advanced Yoga Teacher, Spiritual Director, or Therapist.

YAMAS AND NIYAMAS

PRINCIPLES OF BEING

YOUR OUTER WORLD - YAMAS

Ahimsa - Gentle Love

Satya - Honesty

Asteya - Sharing

Bramacharya - Conscious Intimacy

Aparigraha - Non-Attachment

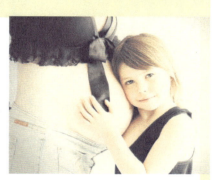

YOUR INNER WORLD - *NIYAMAS*

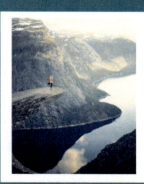

Saucha - Purity

Santosha - Contentment

Svhadhyaya - Self-Study

Ishvara Pranidhana - Surrender to the Universe

Tapas - Self-Discipline

Asana – Physical Yoga Postures

Physical Yoga postures will help you feel more spacious in your body and even relax or energize you. What feels good in your body? What doesn't feel good? Notice and work with where you're at. You'll have an opportunity to practice the Asanas in the next part of the book, Spiritual Bootcamp.

Pranayama – Breathwork

Breathwork, or *pranayama*, will help you utilize the life force energy already within you. One of the great secrets of Yoga is that the mind and the breath are linked, they are on the same spectrum. When you learn to slow and focus your breath, you learn to slow and focus your mind. See Chapter 7: Pranayama Practices.

Pratyahara – Withdrawal of the Senses

Inner awareness and the withdrawal of the senses is a tool we use to let go of the external world and begin to learn more about our own internal landscape. As you learn about yourself, you learn about the part of the universe that exists within you. This tool is helpful in pregnancy and birth as it helps you learn to trust yourself and to let go of external influences. You may hear a negative birth story and this tool will help you turn inwards to encourage and love your own story and let go of someone elses story.

Dharana- Focused Concentration

Focused concentration, a skill that comes with practice, can be used in moments of discomfort or fear. Focusing your eyes on an object or face during birth helps quiet the mind. You can practice this skill by focusing your eyes on a candle for 5-10 minutes. Blinking and blurring vision is okay, just keep your gaze steady.

Dhyana- Meditative Absorption

The key to Meditative Absorption is to notice the space in between your thoughts. The experience of absorption can occur during a meditation, where you get a glimpse of your soul. For some women, myself included, this experience can happen during birth as well. It is very grounding and relaxing to glimpse your deeper self, and can help the body move through its natural urges to hug baby down during contractions.

Samadhi- Oneness

Samadhi and Dhyana are very closely linked. Generally, when one glimpses the soul, there is a realization that we are all one. In this awareness, we remember that we are loved and supported by a power much greater than ourselves. To practice *Samadhi*, lie down and let the awareness of the boundaries of the edges of your body fade away. This practice can be done more easily by bringing your awareness to the oneness of you and your baby. This practice is much easier to do when you are pregnant because the boundaries between you and your baby are blurry. This practice becomes more challenging after baby is born. See more on Oneness, *Samadhi*, in the Chapter 5.

Five

Oneness, Samadhi

The ultimate goal of Yoga, to experience oneness with the universe (*Samadhi*), requires us to be free and boundless. Being free, in the Yogic sense, is to let go of our misguided thinking that leads us to believe that we are separate from the universe.

The truth is, we are one with the universe. So we must let go of the misidentification of the Self with the non-self. We must realize who we truly are.

Pregnancy and motherhood shift us from one identity to another. Since a pregnant woman is already undergoing this shift, it is a good time to remember that these are all external identities and masks over who we truly are: One. Many women have brief insights of this oneness with the universe. Because women are participating so intimately with creation, many will experience that deep knowledge of our unity. However, for many, including myself, this can be shadowed by holding on to our past and even holding on to our expectations of the future.

We hold on to our past when we cannot let go of who we thought we were, even as monumental shifts happen. We hold on to our future when we cannot let go of who we think we should be, instead of realizing who we actually are. And who we are, at the deepest level, is a spark of the universe.

Coming to this realization of oneness allows the pregnant woman's mind and body to be a little more at ease, and to navigate pregnancy, birth, and motherhood with wisdom and calm. This realization is by no means all encompassing, because it happens moment by moment. Some moments you will feel oneness, others you will not. The goal is to practice moving in and out of that state of awareness so that it is easily available to you when you need it during labor and birth. The tools in the next part of the book will help you find your flow with the universe.

PART II

Spiritual Bootcamp – Body, Mind, Spirit

I define "Spiritual Bootcamp" as a mind, body, spirit, experience of facing fears, going out into the unknown, and returning anew. It is a predictable process that unfolds during pregnancy and into motherhood. As with any natural process, we can either work with it or against it.
In Part III, you will learn how to work with the unfolding spiritual journey that you are already experiencing during pregnancy. This guide will take you through mantras for meditation and stilling the mind, yoga postures for physical preparation and comfort, foods for your growing body, and stories for reflection.

Six

15 Minute Yoga Asana Practices for the Body

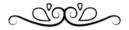

How To Use This Section

Consider the quote in purple while you practice the Yoga sequences on the following page. Every time your mind begins to wander, return your inner dialogue back to the words and ideas of the quote and the theme. Notice how your inner language can change the sensations of the pose. If there are some words that work for you better than others, choose to focus on what works and to let go of what doesn't.

As always, when starting a new exercise program, please consult your physician. Though all of the poses are safe for general pregnancy, throughout all 3 trimesters, please take note of the contraindications for each pose. And if there is a position that causes you any pain, slowly come out of it.

You can do one sequence a day, or combine sequences for longer exercise routines. If you have time, it is nice to sit or lay down after your practice to enjoy a *Savasana* (relaxation pose) and absorb inner stillness.

In the second part of this chapter, you will see 5 Minute Yoga Practices to give you ideas on how to find some more space in your body and mind in just 5 minutes.

It will be helpful to have the following materials:

1) Yoga Mat
   2) A Yoga Block or wide, sturdy water bottle
   3) 2 Yoga Bolsters, or 2 sturdy couch cushions
   4) A throw blanket or towel to sit on
   5) Music
   6) Candle
   7) A sturdy stool or chair

> "To the mind that is still, the whole universe surrenders."
>
> —Lao Tzu

Spirit Birth

15 Minute Yoga Asana Practices for the Body

STILLNESS

AND DECREASE LOW BACK PAIN

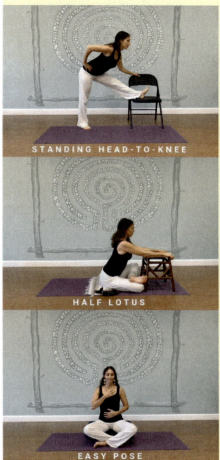

STANDING HEAD-TO-KNEE
STAND TO THE RIGHT OF A CHAIR, TURN TO FACE IT. INHALE AND PLACE YOUR RIGHT HEEL ON THE CHAIR. PAUSE TO SETTLE IN, THEN INHALE AND STRAIGHTEN YOUR LEG. YOU MAY ALREADY FEEL A GENTLE TUG IN YOUR HAMSTRING. IF IT FEELS ACCESSIBLE, EXHALE AND BEGIN TO LEAN YOUR BELLY TO THE INSIDE OF YOUR THIGH. YOUR RIGHT HAND RESTS ON THE BACK OF THE CHAIR, THE LEFT HAND COMES TO THE HIP. PRESS DOWN THROUGH YOUR LEFT FOOT, INHALE AND LIFT UP THROUGH THE HEART. EXHALE AND SOFTEN THE FACE AND SHOULDERS. BRING YOUR AWARENESS TO BABY AS YOU BOW INWARD. STAY IN THIS POSE FOR 5 OR MORE BREATHS. TO COME OUT OF THE POSE, INHALE, PRESSING INTO THE LEFT FOOT AND RAISING THE TORSO BACK TO NEUTRAL. REPEAT ON THE OTHER SIDE.
CONTRAINDICATIONS: FOR ASTHMA, KEEP THE CHIN LIFTED.

HALF LOTUS
SIT ON A BLANKET FACING A STOOL OR CHAIR. CROSS YOUR RIGHT ANKLE IN FRONT OF YOUR LEFT. USE YOUR HANDS TO PULL THE FLESH AWAY FROM YOUR SIT BONES, HELPING TO ROOT THE BODY DOWN. PLACE YOUR RIGHT HAND ON YOUR RIGHT KNEE, AND YOUR LEFT HAND ON YOUR RIGHT FOOT CRADLING THE LEG. ROCK YOUR LEG, BRINGING AWARENESS TO WHERE THE THIGH BONE ENTERS THE HIP SOCKET. ON AN EXHALE SLOWLY LOWER YOUR RIGHT FOOT ONTO YOUR LEFT THIGH. IF YOUR KNEES FEEL PAIN, RELEASE THE FOOT TO THE FLOOR. INHALE AND LENGTHEN THROUGH THE SPINE. IF IT'S ACCESSIBLE, EXHALE AND BEGIN TO BRING BELLY FORWARD AND DOWN, REACHING YOUR ARMS FOR THE SUPPORT IN FRONT OF YOU. YOU MAY KEEP YOUR NECK LONG OR LET IT HANG. AWARENESS FOCUSES ON THE PLACE WHERE PELVIS AND EARTH CONNECT.
CONTRAINDICATIONS: KNEE OR ANKLE INJURY.

EASY POSE
SIT CROSS-LEGGED ON THE FLOOR, WITH THE RIGHT ANKLE IN FRONT. FOR EXTRA SUPPORT, SIT ON A BOLSTER OR FOLDED BLANKET. LET YOUR HIPS BE HEAVY AND THE CROWN OF YOUR HEAD REACH TOWARD THE SKY. BRING YOUR AWARENESS TO YOUR HEART AND YOUR WOMB. BREATHE. REPEAT ON THE OTHER SIDE.
CONTRAINDICATIONS: FOR KNEE INJURY, USE CAUTION

Spirit Birth

> "Have patience with all things, but first of all with yourself."
> —Saint Francis de Sales

Spirit Birth

15 Minute Yoga Asana Practices for the Body

PATIENCE
AND DECREASE SHOULDER PAIN

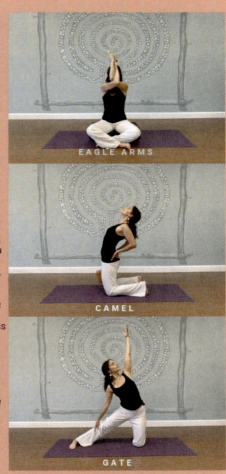

EAGLE ARMS
SIT ON THE FLOOR OR A CHAIR, INHALE AND OPEN YOUR ARMS WIDE. EXHALE, WRAP YOUR ARMS AROUND YOURSELF, RIGHT ARM ON TOP. IF THIS FEELS GOOD, STAY HERE. TO GO DEEPER, LIFT THE FOREARMS VERTICALLY, PRESSING THE BACKS OF THE HANDS TOGETHER IN FRONT OF THE HEAD, OR, WRAP THE PALMS AROUND AND PRESS TOGETHER. INHALE AND REACH THROUGH THE CROWN OF YOUR HEAD, EXHALE AND SOFTEN THE TOPS OF THE SHOULDERS. STAY HERE FOR 5 OR MORE BREATHS. ON AN EXHALE, UNWIND THE ARMS. REPEAT ON THE OTHER SIDE.
CONTRAINDICATIONS: FOR SHOULDER INJURY, USE CAUTION

CAMEL
KNEEL, KNEES UNDER HIP JOINTS. TOES TUCK, HEELS LIFT. HOLD A BLOCK BETWEEN THE THIGHS, AND PRESS THE PUBIC BONE FORWARD. LENGTHEN YOUR ABDOMEN UPWARD, OUT OF THE PELVIC BOWL, PALMS TO LOW BACK, FINGERS FACE DOWN. PRESS THE HEELS OF YOUR HANDS INTO THE TOP OF THE HIP-BONES ON EITHER SIDE. USE THE SUPPORT OF YOUR HANDS TO LIFT AND OPEN YOUR HEART. PELVIS FORWARD, LEAN BACK INTO THE SUPPORT OF YOUR HANDS. BRING YOUR AWARENESS TO THE STRENGTH AND RECEPTIVITY OF THE HEART. STAY HERE FOR 3-10 BREATHS. TO COME OUT OF THE POSE, THE HEAD COMES UP LAST. SO BRING THE HIPS IN LINE, THEN THE HEART, AND FINALLY THE HEAD.
CONTRAINDICATIONS: HIGH OR LOW BLOOD PRESSURE; MIGRAINE; INSOMNIA; OR SERIOUS LOW BACK OR NECK INJURY.

GATE
FROM HIGH KNEES, EXTEND YOUR RIGHT LEG OUT TO THE RIGHT. IF YOUR LEFT KNEE FEELS TENDER, PLACE A BLANKET UNDER THE KNEE. INHALE, OPEN YOUR ARMS OUT LIKE WINGS. EXHALE AS YOU REACH TOWARD YOUR RIGHT TOES, THEN LOWER YOUR RIGHT HAND DOWN TO YOUR SHIN OR THIGH. THE LEFT ARM REACHES STRAIGHT UP. INHALE AND LIFT THROUGH THE RIGHT SIDE OF THE BODY, EXHALE AND SOFTEN THROUGH THE LEFT SIDE OF THE BODY. YOUR GAZE CAN TURN UP OR DOWN. TO COME OUT OF THE POSE, INHALE AND COME UP TO A NEUTRAL SPINE. EXHALE AND RELEASE THE LEG TO HIGH KNEES. REPEAT ON THE OTHER SIDE.
CONTRAINDICATIONS: FOR KNEE, HIP, LOW BACK, AND NECK INJURY, USE CAUTION.

Spirit Birth

"Whenever you accept what is, something deeper emerges than what is. So, you can be trapped in the most painful dilemma, external or internal, the most painful feelings or situation, and the moment you accept what is, you go beyond it, you transcend it...Even if you feel hatred, the moment you accept that this is what you feel, you transcend it. It may still be there, but suddenly you are at a deeper place where it doesn't matter that much anymore."

-Eckart Tolle

Spirit Birth

15 Minute Yoga Asana Practices for the Body

ACCEPTANCE
AND DECREASE HIP PAIN

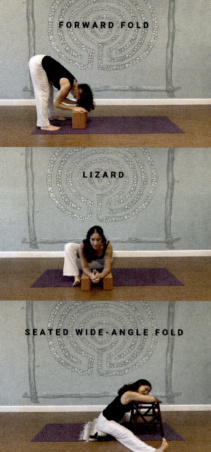

FORWARD FOLD
STAND ON YOUR MAT WITH BLOCKS NEXT TO YOUR FEET. OPEN YOUR FEET A LITTLE WIDER THAN YOUR HIPS. INHALE AND REACH YOUR ARMS UP TO THE SKY. EXHALE, BEND FORWARD, BRINGING BELLY TOWARD THE THIGHS. INHALE AND TAKE YOUR HANDS TO THE BLOCKS, LIFTING THE TORSO UP SLIGHTLY, GETTING LENGTH IN THE SPINE. EXHALE SOFTEN YOUR BELLY, HEART, AND HEAD FORWARD. KEEP YOUR HANDS FIRM ON THE BLOCKS. ENJOY FOR 5-10 BREATHS. IF YOU FEEL DIZZY OR HAVE LOW BACK PAIN, BEND YOUR KNEES. TO COME OUT OF THE POSE, SQUEEZE YOUR THIGHS TOGETHER, INHALE AND RISE UP TO STANDING.
CONTRAINDICATIONS: FOR BACK INJURY, HIGH OR LOW BLOOD PRESSURE, BEND KNEES OR COME HALF-WAY UP

LIZARD
FROM HANDS AND KNEES. INHALE AND BRING YOUR RIGHT FOOT FORWARD TO THE OUTER RIGHT EDGE OF YOUR MAT. PLACE YOUR BLOCKS TO THE INSIDE OF THE RIGHT FOOT. EXHALE AND BEGIN TO LOWER YOUR BELLY AND CHEST DOWN, LEANING INTO THE BLOCKS. IF IT'S ACCESSIBLE, COME DOWN ONTO YOUR FOREARMS. IF THIS DOESN'T FEEL COMFORTABLE, STRAIGHTEN YOUR ARMS AND EVEN RAISE YOUR BLOCKS TO THE NEXT HEIGHT. PAUSE. ON YOUR NEXT INHALATION, LIFT THE BIG-TOE SIDE OF THE RIGHT FOOT OFF THE MAT, PRESSING INTO THE PINKY-TOE SIDE OF THE FOOT. GAZE IS SLIGHTLY FORWARD. DRAW YOUR AWARENESS DOWN TO YOUR HIPS AND PELVIS AS THEY RELEASE, LITTLE BY LITTLE. STAY HERE FOR 3-10 BREATHS. TO COME OUT OF THE POSE, INHALE AND PRESS THE WHOLE RIGHT FOOT INTO THE MAT, ARMS STRAIGHTEN. EXHALE AND RELEASE THE LEG BACK TO HANDS AND KNEES. REPEAT ON THE OTHER SIDE.
CONTRAINDICATIONS: HIP AND KNEE INJURY

SEATED WIDE-ANGLE FOLD
SIT ON A BLANKET FACING YOUR STOOL, LEGS OPEN WIDE. TOES AND KNEES POINT UP. IF THIS IS TOO INTENSE, ADD ANOTHER BLANKET OR BOLSTER UNDER YOUR HIPS. INHALE AND REACH YOUR ARMS TOWARD THE SKY. EXHALE AND BRING BELLY FORWARD AS YOUR ARMS REACH FOR THE STOOL. REST YOUR HEAD ON YOUR HANDS IF IT IS COMFORTABLE. AS YOU SETTLE INTO THIS POSE, ALLOW YOUR HIPS TO BE HEAVY AND YOUR FACE TO BE SOFT. BRING YOUR AWARENESS TO YOUR PELVIS AND BREATHE. STAY HERE FOR 5 OR MORE BREATHS.
CONTRAINDICATIONS: FOR LOW BACK INJURY, SIT UP HIGHER ON A FOLDED BLANKET AND LEAN THE TORSO ONLY SLIGHTLY FORWARD.

Spirit Birth

> "Live from the heart of yourself. Seek to be whole, not perfect."
> -Oprah

Spirit Birth

15 Minute Yoga Asana Practices for the Body

STRENGTH
AND REDUCE ANXIETY

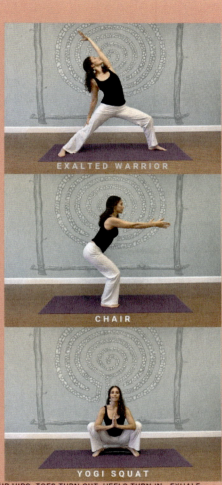

EXALTED WARRIOR

FROM STANDING, STEP YOUR LEGS WIDE. TURN YOUR RIGHT TOES TOWARD THE FRONT OF YOUR MAT, AND YOUR LEFT FOOT PARALLEL TO THE BACK OF THE MAT. IF YOU FEEL UNSTEADY, STEP YOUR RIGHT FOOT TOWARD THE RIGHT EDGE OF THE MAT. EXHALE AND BEND THE RIGHT KNEE. INHALE AND OPEN THE ARMS OUT WIDE, LIKE WINGS. THE GAZE TURNS TOWARD THE RIGHT HAND. INHALE AND LIFT THE RIGHT ARM UP AS THE LEFT HAND COMES TO THE LEFT THIGH. EXHALE AND LEAN THE HEAD AND CHEST BACK SLIGHTLY. TO COME OUT OF THE POSE, INHALE THE ARMS BACK TO NEUTRAL AND STRAIGHTEN THE FRONT LEG. REPEAT ON THE OTHER SIDE.
CONTRAINDICATIONS: FOR KNEE, HIP, LOW BACK, OR NECK INJURY, USE CAUTION

CHAIR

STANDING WITH FEET A LITTLE WIDER THAN HIP-WIDTH DISTANCE APART, REACH YOUR ARMS FORWARD. HUG YOUR THIGHS TOWARDS ONE ANOTHER, INVITING YOUR THIGH MUSCLES TO ENGAGE STRONGLY. AS YOU EXHALE, BEND YOUR KNEES, AS IF SITTING IN A CHAIR. LOWER YOUR HIPS UNTIL YOU FEEL YOUR LEGS WORKING. PRESS YOUR PUBIC BONE FORWARD, LENGTHENING THE LOWER BACK. FOCUS YOUR AWARENESS ON YOUR WOMB SPACE. SEND LOVE TO YOUR BABY AS YOU SOFTEN YOUR FACE AND SHOULDERS. BREATHE. STAY HERE ANYWHERE FROM 10 SECONDS- 2 MINUTES. THEN INHALE AND SLOWLY STRAIGHTEN YOUR LEGS, RELEASING YOUR ARMS TO YOUR SIDE. VARIATIONS: STRAIGHTEN YOUR ARMS OVER HEAD, OR HOLD A BLOCK BETWEEN THE THIGHS.
CONTRAINDICATIONS: KNEE INJURY, HEADACHE, INSOMNIA, LOW BLOOD PRESSURE.

YOGI SQUAT

FROM STANDING, OPEN YOUR FEET WIDER THAN YOUR HIPS. TOES TURN OUT, HEELS TURN IN. EXHALE, BEND THE KNEES, LOWER THE HIPS DOWNWARD. OPTIONS: TAKE A BLANKET UNDER YOUR HEELS, OR A BLOCK UNDER YOUR BUTTOCKS. EXHALE AND BRING PALMS TOGETHER AT THE HEART. ELBOWS PRESS OUT AGAINST THE KNEES. KNEES PRESS BACK ON THE ELBOWS. INHALE AND LIFT YOUR HEART. EXHALE, LET YOUR HIPS BE HEAVY. BRING YOUR AWARENESS TO YOUR WOMB AND PELVIS. VISUALIZE WOMEN WHO HAVE BIRTHED BEFORE YOU ARE SMILING AT YOU. BREATHE. STAY HERE FOR 1-2 MINUTES. TO COME OUT, INHALE, LEAN FORWARD AND STRAIGHTEN THE LEGS TO COME BACK UP TO STANDING.
CONTRAINDICATIONS: AFTER 36 WEEKS, BABY MUST BE HEAD DOWN TO GO INTO THE DEEP VERSION OF THIS POSE. FOR OBSTRUCTIONS (PLACENTA PREVIA) SIT ON TWO BLOCKS. FOR HIP AND KNEE INJURY, USE CAUTION.

Spirit Birth

> "Authenticity is a collection of choices that we have to make everyday. It's about the choice to show up and be real. The choice to let our true selves be seen."
>
> -Brene Brown

Spirit Birth

15 Minute Yoga Asana Practices for the Body

BALANCE
AND DECREASE ANGER

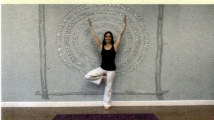
TREE

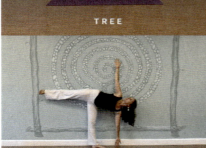
HALF MOON

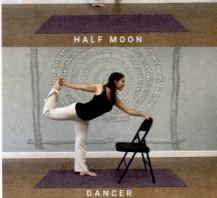
DANCER

TREE AT THE WALL
STAND WITH YOUR BACK TO THE WALL, ABOUT 2 INCHES AWAY. INHALE AND ELONGATE YOUR NECK, EXHALE AND PRESS DOWN THROUGH YOUR FEET. LET YOUR EYES SETTLE ON A SPOT ON THE FLOOR IN FRONT OF YOU. INHALE AND BEND YOUR RIGHT KNEE, OPENING IT OUT TO YOUR SIDE, AND PLACING THE FOOT ON THE ANKLE, THE SHIN, OR THE THIGH, ABOVE THE KNEE. LEAN INTO THE WALL, AS NEEDED. HANDS CAN COME TO YOUR HEART OR REACH OVERHEAD. FOCUS YOUR AWARENESS ON BRINGING LENGTH FROM THE BOTTOM OF YOUR SPINE ALL THE WAY INTO THE HEAD. STAY HERE FOR 10 BREATHS OR MORE. TO COME OUT OF THE POSE, EXHALE, RELEASE YOUR KNEE FORWARD AND LOWER THE FOOT TO THE GROUND. REPEAT ON THE LEFT SIDE.
CONTRAINDICATIONS: FOR POOR BALANCE, STAY LEANING AGAINST THE WALL.

HALF MOON AT THE WALL
STAND AT THE WALL, WITH 3 INCHES OF SPACE BETWEEN YOUR FEET AND THE WALL. TURN YOUR RIGHT TOES PARALLEL TO THE WALL. EXHALE, LOOK DOWN AND BEGIN TO REACH YOUR RIGHT HAND TOWARD THE FLOOR OR A BLOCK. LEAN INTO THE WALL WHEN YOU NEED EXTRA SUPPORT. INHALE AND LIFT THE LEFT ARM STRAIGHT UP, CREATING ONE LONG LINE FROM YOUR BOTTOM ARM TO YOUR TOP. TURN YOUR GAZE UP OR DOWN, DEPENDING ON YOUR PREFERENCE. THE LEFT HIP STACKS ON TOP OF THE RIGHT, OPENING THE PELVIS SLIGHTLY. INHALE AND PRESS OUT THROUGH THE HEEL OF YOUR LEFT FOOT. STAY FOR 5 OR MORE BREATHS. TO COME OUT OF THE POSE, TURN YOUR GAZE DOWN AND LEAN INTO THE WALL BEHIND YOU. INHALE AS YOU PRESS INTO YOUR RIGHT LEG AND RETURN THE TORSO TO A NEUTRAL POSITION. REPEAT ON THE OTHER SIDE.
CONTRAINDICATIONS: HEADACHE, LOW BLOOD PRESSURE

DANCER
STAND FACING A CHAIR OR TABLE. GAZE AT THE FLOOR, ABOUT 3 FEET AHEAD. AS YOU INHALE, BEND YOUR RIGHT KNEE, GRASP YOUR RIGHT FOOT WITH YOUR RIGHT HAND. PAUSE. INHALE AND LIFT YOUR LEFT ARM, LENGTHEN THE SPINE. EXHALE, BOW FORWARD REACHING YOUR LEFT HAND TO THE CHAIR OR TABLE. PRESS YOUR RIGHT FOOT INTO YOUR HAND, KICK THE HEEL AWAY FROM THE BUTTOCK, AND OPEN THE FRONT RIGHT HIP. THE RIGHT SHOULDER BLADE FLOATS BACK, OPENING THE HEART. BRING YOUR AWARENESS TO THE OPENING OF THE FRONT OF YOUR BODY, AND THE STRENGTH OF YOUR BACK BODY. STAY HERE FOR 5+ BREATHS. TO COME OUT, SLOWLY RELEASE THE FOOT AND COME INTO A FORWARD FOLD USING THE CHAIR OR TABLE. REPEAT ON THE LEFT SIDE.
CONTRAINDICATIONS: KNEE INJURY, HIGH OR LOW BLOOD PRESSURE, MIGRAINE, SERIOUS LOW BACK OR NECK INJURY.

Spirit Birth

Seven

5 Minute Yoga Practices

How To Use This Section

The following yoga poses are ways to integrate Yoga in small spurts throughout the day. Whether you're waiting for the kettle to boil or for your older child to fall asleep, you can integrate these poses and mental concepts. You may also do these poses in sequential order to enjoy a 30 minute practice.

Use each pose's theme as a focal point for your mind, repeating the word or words silently in your mind as you settle into your pose. As your mind begins to wander, bring it back to the theme.

It will be helpful to have the following materials:

1) Yoga Mat
   2) A Yoga Block or wide, sturdy water bottle
   3) 2 Yoga Bolsters, or 2 sturdy couch cushions
   4) A throw blanket or towel to sit on
   5) Music
   6) Candle

7) A sturdy stool or chair

5 Minute Yoga Practices

RECEIVE
EVERYTHING IS OKAY

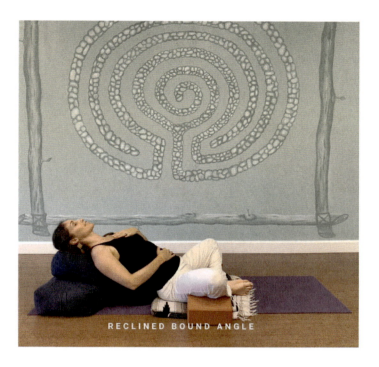

RECLINED BOUND ANGLE

RECLINED BOUND ANGLE

TAKE TWO LARGE BOLSTERS PERPENDICULAR TO ONE ANOTHER, CREATING A RAMP WITH THE TOP BOLSTER, ANGLED DOWN TOWARDS THE MIDDLE OF THE MAT. PLACE A BLANKET UP AGAINST THE BOTTOM OF THE RAMP, WHERE IT MEETS THE MAT.
SIT ON THE BLANKET WITH THE BUTTOCKS UP AGAINST THE BOTTOM OF THE RAMP. BRING THE BOTTOMS OF THE FEET TOGETHER AND ALLOW THE KNEES TO OPEN SOFTLY. YOU MAY SUPPORT THE OUTSIDE OF YOUR KNEES WITH BLOCKS IF YOU LIKE. USING THE STRENGTH OF YOUR ARMS, LOWER YOURSELF DOWN ONTO THE BOLSTER. TAKE ONE HAND TO YOUR WOMB, ONE HAND TO YOUR HEART.
PRESS THE BELLY OUT AS YOU DRAW IN YOUR BREATH. PULL THE BELLY IN AS YOU BREATH OUT. LET YOUR BREATH SLOW. AFTER A FEW CONSCIOUS BREATHS, BEGIN TO NOTICE THE TRANSITION FROM INHALE TO EXHALE. NOTICE IF THERE IS A HESITATION AS YOU SWITCH FROM ONE TO THE OTHER, AND BEGIN TO BRING AWARENESS TO THAT MOMENT, ALLOWING THE INHALE AND THE EXHALE TO BEGIN TO FLOW IN A GRACEFUL CYCLE, WHERE ONE BECOMES THE OTHER.

Spirit Birth

5 Minute Yoga Practices

SPACIOUSNESS
IN THE PRESENT MOMENT

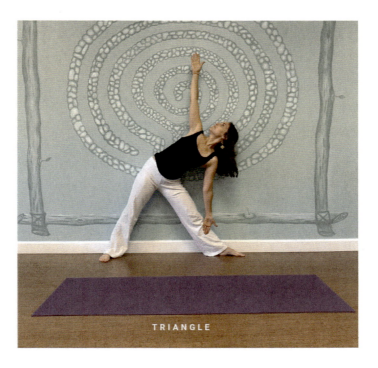

TRIANGLE

TRIANGLE

STAND WITH YOUR BACK TO THE WALL, ABOUT 2 INCHES AWAY. OPEN YOUR LEGS WIDE, TURNING YOUR RIGHT TOES TOWARD THE RIGHT, YOUR LEFT TOES FACING FORWARD. OPEN YOUR ARMS OUT WIDE, PALMS TURN DOWN. INHALE AND REACH TOWARD THE RIGHT SIDE OF THE ROOM, LEANING THAT DIRECTION WITH THE TORSO. EXHALE AND RELEASE YOUR RIGHT HAND DOWN TOWARD THE FLOOR, SHIN, OR THIGH. THE LEFT ARM REACHES STRAIGHT UP, AS THE RIGHT ARM REACHES STRAIGHT DOWN. GAZE TURNS UP OR DOWN, WHICHEVER IS MORE COMFORTABLE TO YOU. YOU CAN ALLOW YOUR BODY TO LEAN INTO THE WALL BEHIND YOU, OR STAY STANDING. BRING YOUR AWARENESS TO THE INNER THIGHS AS THEY STRETCH. NOTICE THE GENTLE STRETCH IN YOUR LEFT HIP AND LOW BACK. BREATHE. STAY HERE FOR 3-10 BREATHS. TO COME OUT OF THE POSE, INHALE AND RETURN TO STANDING. REPEAT ON THE OTHER SIDE. CONTRAINDICATIONS: FOR HIP AND LOW BACK INJURY, USE CAUTION.

Spirit Birth

5 Minute Yoga Practices

COMMUNICATE
LISTEN AND SPEAK

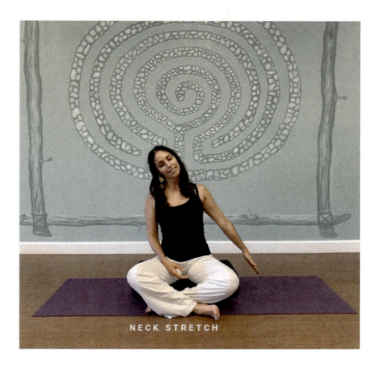

NECK STRETCH

SITTING ON A BOLSTER OR CHAIR, INHALE AND LENGTHEN THROUGH THE CROWN OF THE HEAD. AS YOU EXHALE, SOFTEN THE SHOULDERS. TAKE YOUR RIGHT ARM TO YOUR SIDE, AND THE LEFT HAND CAN REST COMFORTABLY IN YOUR LAP. INHALE AND STRAIGHTEN THE FINGERS, MOVING THE PALM OF THE HAND AWAY FROM THE HIPS ABOUT A FOOT. IMAGINE YOU ARE TRYING TO PUSH YOUR FINGERS INTO THE SAND, PRESSING DOWN AND AWAY FROM YOU. AS YOU EXHALE, SLOWLY RELEASE THE HEAD TOWARD THE LEFT SHOULDER. LEAN YOUR HEAD BACK INTO AN IMAGINARY HEADREST AND OPEN THROUGH THE FRONT OF THE SHOULDER. STAY HERE FOR 5 OR MORE BREATHS. TO COME OUT OF THE POSE, INHALE AND LIFT THE HEAD, RELEASING THE ARM. REPEAT ON THE OTHER SIDE
CONTRAINDICATIONS: FOR NECK OR SHOULDER INJURY, USE CAUTION.

Spirit Birth

5 Minute Yoga Practices

YES, UNIVERSE
THANK YOU

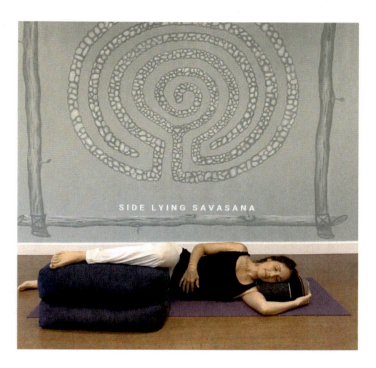

SIDE LYING SAVASANA

LIE ON YOUR LEFT SIDE, WITH YOUR HEAD SUPPORTED BY A PILLOW OR FOLDED BLANKET. SUPPORT YOUR TOP KNEE AND FOOT ON ONE OR TWO BOLSTERS. STRAIGHTEN YOUR BOTTOM LEG.
LET THE SIDE OF YOUR BODY MELT WITH EVERY EXHALATION. BRING YOUR AWARENESS TO YOUR BABY AND BREATHE. ALLOW YOUR THOUGHTS TO FLOAT AWAY AS YOU OBSERVE YOUR BREATH. STAY HERE FOR 3-10 MINUTES. TO COME OUT OF THE POSE, SLIDE THE BOLSTERS AWAY. PRESS YOUR RIGHT HAND INTO THE MAT AND LIFT YOUR TORSO UPRIGHT.

Spirit Birth

5 Minute Yoga Practices

RHYTHM, RITUAL, RELAXATION
TOOLS FOR LABOR

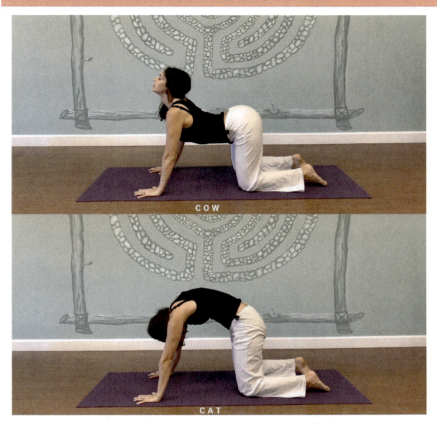

CAT COW

COME TO HANDS AND KNEES, KNEES A LITTLE WIDER THAN YOUR HIPS, MAKING ROOM FOR BABY. HANDS ARE UNDER THE SHOULDER JOINTS. AS YOU EXHALE, PRESS INTO YOUR HANDS AND KNEES, ROUND YOUR SPINE UPWARD TOWARD THE SKY, TUCK YOUR CHIN IN TOWARD YOUR CHEST, AND YOUR TAILBONE POINTS TOWARD THE EARTH. BRING YOUR AWARENESS TO YOUR SOLAR PLEXUS AS YOU LENGTHEN THE SPINE. LET IN YOUR INHALE TAKE YOU OUT OF THE POSE TO A NEUTRAL SPINE. AS YOU INHALE, LOWER YOUR BELLY WHILE LIFTING YOUR HEAD AND TAILBONE. AS YOU EXHALE RELEASE TO CAT. LET YOUR BREATH GUIDE YOU UNTIL YOU FIND YOUR RHYTHM.
CONTRAINDICATIONS: FOR TENDERNESS ON THE BELLY, DO NOT ARCH THE LOW-BACK, RATHER, FOCUS ON LIFTING THE HEAD. FOR NECK INJURIES OR PAIN, KEEP THE HEAD IN LINE WITH THE TORSO.

Spirit Birth

5 Minute Yoga Practices

THE SUBTLE
LAYERS OF THE SELF

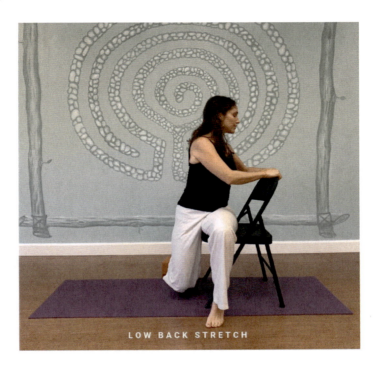

LOW BACK STRETCH

LOW BACK STRETCH

SIT ON A STURDY CHAIR, WITH YOUR FEET ON THE GROUND. TURN TOWARD THE LEFT, SITTING ON YOUR LIFT HIP, AND LETTING YOUR RIGHT HIP HANG OFF THE EDGE OF THE CHAIR. PRESS INTO YOUR LEFT FOOT AND HOLD ON TO THE BACK OF THE CHAIR.
BEND YOUR RIGHT KNEE AND TAKE YOUR FOOT BEHIND YOU. LET YOUR RIGHT LEG BE HEAVY, AS IF SOMEONE WERE TAKING THEIR HANDS TO YOUR THIGH AND GENTLY TUGGING IT DOWNWARD. TURN TOWARD THE BACK OF THE CHAIR, PLACING BOTH HANDS ON THE BACK OF THE CHAIR.
BRING YOUR AWARENESS TO WHERE YOUR HIPS ARE SUPPORTED BY THE CHAIR. NOTICE THE SUBTLE RELEASE OF THE LOW BACK. BREATHE. STAY HERE FOR 5 OR MORE BREATHS.
ON AN INHALE, PLEASE TURN AND FACE FORWARD. REPEAT THIS POSE ON THE OTHER SIDE.

Eight

Pranayama Practices for the Breath

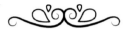

Your breath will naturally pick up as your body works harder. It will naturally slow down as your body calms. But one of the great secrets of yoga and meditation is that we can also consciously change our breath, and thus change our body and mind. You can combine some of these *pranayama* practices with *asanas* from Chapters 6 and 7.

* * *

Breath Awareness- For Calm

Sit comfortably or lie down. If you can, let someone calmly read this aloud as you close your eyes.

Notice the temperature of the breath as you inhale through the nose. Notice the temperature of the breath as you exhale through the nose. On your next inhale, notice where in your body fills with breath. As you exhale, notice your body letting go. Continue to notice your body breathing. Your thoughts continue to slip away as your awareness settles in on your beautiful breath, receiving and returning. Continue for 1-15 minutes.

Conscious Relaxation- For Relief

Sit comfortably or lie down. If you can, let someone calmly read this aloud as you close your eyes.

Bring your awareness to your feet, to the spaces in between your toes. As you exhale, relax and release this space. Bring your awareness and relaxation to:

Your shins and calves, relax and release.
Your thighs become heavy with relaxation.
Hips and low back are releasing.
The womb softens, baby is safe and warm.
The muscles in between your ribs relax.
Armpits release.
Arm bones are heavy with relaxation.
Palms release, finger nail beds let go.
Back of the throat softens.
Back of the tongue releases.
Muscles around the eyes let go.

And the spaces in between the hairs on the top of your head melt like butter as your whole body moves into conscious relaxation.

Ujjayi Breathing (Victorious Breath) For Strength

Sit comfortably or lie down. Inhale and exhale through the nose, consciously slowing the breath, little by little. Begin to make the sound of the ocean waves with your breath, hugging the back of your throat. Continue breathing in this way for 5 minutes.

*Note: if you are taking hypnobirthing classes, this type of breathing might not be recommended.

Focus on the Exhale- For Pushing

Take a short inhale through the nose, and release a long exhale through pursed lips. Focus on the exhalation: Press all of the breath out, making room for new breath. Practice for 1 minute.

Panting- For Baby Crowning During Delivery

Stick out your tongue like a dog, inhale and exhale like a panting dog. Practice for 1 minute.

Nine

Mantras and Ideas for the Mind

In this section, each theme is discussed and a personal story shared. You can read these in order, or just skip to the theme that is calling you today. Once you have read the story and discussion, take 1-5 minutes to sit silently and repeat the mantra in your mind. It is helpful to practice these mantras regularly to help prepare the mind for birth.

***

Time

It takes time for the cervix to open, time for baby to move down. During labor, you might question, "How much time will this take?".

It takes time to become a mother. It takes time to become wise, to let wisdom repeat itself until we don't have to think about it anymore- It takes time to make a habit out of being wise. It takes time for children to gain new skills. It takes time for us to see them as they truly are.

And yet, once these moments pass, we say, "It all goes by so quickly."

It takes time to make a habit of being wise.

Yoga aims to liberate the self from cycles of time, so that one can experience linear, chronological time, and the stillness of deep time at once. Deep time refers to those moments where we think to ourselves, "It doesn't get any better than this," or "Oh, yes, I get it." As Richard Rohr says, "...where time comes to a fullness, and the dots connect" (*in conversation with Krista Tippett, April 2017*). How can we move from the linear time of clocks and calendars to the deep time of stillness and expansiveness? In birth and motherhood, we can engage our "contemplative mind"(*Rohr*), consider what really matters, what we value, and encounter stress and triumphs with the same perspective.

As you become present with the moments in your life, letting go of the past and the future, your body will begin to feel more at ease. To become present, notice the details of a moment, like the sounds, the sensations, or the memories that arise. Considering time and this mantra during pregnancy helps you prepare for labor by learning to be present now, so that you can be present in your birth.

MANTRA (repeat silently or aloud): *I let time come to its fullness.*

Leaning In To Discomfort

It's a cold fall day in San Diego and my kids are dripping snot. I start to feel my own terrible sore throat coming on. "Oh no!" I think. I have so much to do today, the house is a mess and I don't know how I'm going to get everything done. But, I decide I'll just truck on and make it work. I'm scrubbing the counters, my 3yo is screaming at my 1yo to stop stealing her toys. My head is pounding and terror sets in: How am I going to manage the *whole* day? It's barely 9am.

I make a tent under the dining table and put some toys in there, hoping the girls will stay mellow while I finish mopping. But, I am out of energy, and the baby is pulling the sheets down, toppling over the tent, and sending my 3yo into fits anger.

I am stuck, I'm tired, and I feel helpless. Instead of trying to ignore the discomfort and continue on with my plans for the day unhindered, I decide to lean into the discomfort. I put the mop down, pick the baby up, grab a toy stethyscope and say, "I'm sick, let's play doctor."

The girls are unexpectedly thrilled. They bubble the whole way upstairs. The game is sweet and tender, while of course, short-lasted. Their sniffling bodies grow tired quickly, and as we are already in the bed, they snuggle up and listen to me read softly. Before I know it, they are both fast asleep. I doze off with my two little loves snuggled up close. Everything is good.

I leaned into my discomfor. I let myself be sick, and that feeling guided me towards what needed to happen that day, for my kids, and for me.

...Sometimes the only way out, is through.

Leaning in to the discomfort works in a lot of ways, especially in birth. When a birthing woman leans in to the contractions rather than pulling away from them, her body is able to do the work of moving baby down more easily. Leaning in to contractions helps the cervix to dilate.

Sometimes our bodies and our children only respond when we lean in to the discomfort instead of pulling away; sometimes the only way out is through.

MANTRA: *Sometimes the only way out is through.*

Embracing Support

In general, when it comes to birth, it's helpful to have support like a doula, doctor, and/or midwife. Who are your team?

Feeling safe and trusting requires that the people you work with have integrity and reliability.

If you are on this part of your journey, you may find yourself considering your current relationships. Who do you rely on? Who do you shy away from? Who makes you feel strong, who makes you feel weak? No answer is correct, it's all observations. As you explore the sensations of your body in answer to these questions, notice what comes up for you. If there are actions that need to be taken or areas that you need to explore more, allow yourself to explore these.

Who is your team?

Close your eyes and imagine yourself at your birth if you are pregnant, or if your child is out of your womb and you are looking for a caregiver, imagine your child is getting ready for his/her nap. What kind of presence do you need? Think of areas where you or your child struggle, and consider what would balance this aspect of yourself.
MANTRA: I am held.

Bringing You Peace

I had both my babies in a hospital. And both times, arriving at the hospital slowed my labor. The female body needs to feel comfortable in order to access the kind of intimacy necessary to relax into the contractions and allow labor to progress. But for most women who are giving birth in a hospital, there is a feeling of discomfort and fear as she enters a hospital. Even women giving birth at home experience this for a short period when the midwives arrive, labor slows for 20-30 minutes until the woman adjusts.

In order to prepare for this in birth and in life, set up visual, auditory, or scent cues for yourself. Whenever you are feeling relaxed, light a candle, look at a calming image, or enjoy a scent. Do this when you are already relaxed. Practice doing this daily or weekly. Eventually, you will have created a neural pathway that allows this image, melody, or smell to remind you of the feelings of relaxation and comfort. You can use these cues when you are not relaxed to help cue your body to let go.

The following mantra you can say aloud or silently when you are feeling relaxed to remind you of the physical and spiritual connection you and your baby share.

MANTRA: *Breathe into the womb-heart connection.*

Adjusting the Language of Birth and Motherhood

The social scientist Dr. Ellen Langer, studies the way humans' perceptions and ways of describing situations can influence their health. She did this research with nurses who were trying to lose weight, as well as elderly men who wanted to feel young again. Each study shows that the language of thoughts affect the physical body. Nurses who started to use the word "exercise" to describe their day at the hospital, moving from patient to patient, actually lost more weight.

This same technique is used in birth. Instead of saying "contractions hurt," a woman can say "my body is working hard," or, "My body is hugging baby down," or, "My body is opening." Pain has the connotation that something is wrong. We experience pain when we cut our finger or drop something on our toe. The sensation of a baby being born is not wrong, so we can use a change in language to help us adjust our minds and potentially have better outcomes.

Language can affect how we birth and also how we raise our children. Using the word "Parenting" rather than "disciplining", or "engaging" rather than "teaching," can help frame our minds and bodies in a way that is more productive and healthier. In *The Genius In Every Child*, by Rick Ackerly, he offers different ways of looking at common words we use around parenting. For example the word 'mistake'."A mistake is simply an opportunity to make another decision. The trick is knowing when and how to change your mind." **MANTRA: *I'm making room for*** baby.

Mothering the Mother

How do we teach our children the importance of self-love and self-care? By loving and caring for ourselves. It was a few weeks into motherhood, and I wished someone would just comfort me the way I was taking care of my child. I wished to be held and rocked in someone's arms. I was tired, overwhelmed, and uncertain, and I knew that I just needed to be reminded that everything was okay.

Well, even though my mother lives 10 minutes away, it wasn't a good time to ask for help. So I began to remember my mother's gentle touch as she would stroke the back of my shoulders. I took a hand to my back and began to gently stroke my own back. Little by little I began to relax and let go.

Abhyanga self massage is another way to provide the nurturing, motherly love you have for your baby to yourself. And furthermore, massage in general has been shown to reduce the effects of depression and lessen the levels of the stress hormone, cortisol, by 31% (Hou, 2010). Use a food-grade oil to circularly massage your joints, and stroke the straight areas of your body, spending extra time on the hands and feet, as well as any areas that are sore.

Say yes to support. Whether it's to supporting yourself, or someone else offering you support during pregnancy and in the postpartum period. If it helps you, say yes.

MANTRA: *I say "Yes" to what I need.*

The Intimate Process

Have you heard of the book *Emotional Intelligence* by Daniel Goleman? This groundbreaking book on redefining "what it means to be smart" has helped guide people into understanding and working with their subtle emotional self.

With hormones amplifying emotions, sometimes the emotional self is not so subtle. But I believe this is for a purpose. Pregnancy gives women an opportunity to practice emotional intelligence, in preparation for motherhood. As mothers, we will be the emotion coaches of our children, helping them to understand their emotions, learn limits, and strategize solutions. But in order for us to be able to provide this support, we must acknowledge our own emotions. This gives us the ability to empathize with our children.

Emotions are subtle, and sometimes unexpected. For example, "Lucy" is excited about being a mom, and yet there's a nagging sadness inside her. She says to herself, "I shouldn't feel sad," disconnecting herself from her experience. A week later, she sees her best friend, and starts crying uncontrollably, not knowing why. She says it's just hormones, but she still doesn't understand why she feels so sad.

What would have happened differently if "Lucy" hadn't told herself not to feel sad? How might the awareness of her subtle inner sensations have guided her? Maybe she was sad because her mother lived far away and in exploring that sensation, she might have decided to accept her mother's offer to come stay with her for the weeks following delivery. Subtle emotions can guide us toward unexpected solutions. And as we navigate our own emotional roller coasters, we are preparing to guide our children on their own emotional journeys.

MANTRA: *I honor where my emotions come from.*

The Throat Mirrors the Birth Canal

When I was pregnant with my first child, I wasn't sure if I was going to be a good mom. I was excited, of course, but there was a lot of responsibility and I was feeling overwhelmed. I felt ashamed that I was having these feelings and so I didn't say anything to my husband, or to anyone. I kept my mouth shut, and didn't even allow myself to think about it and explore where these feelings were coming from.

When my water broke and I didn't go in to labor, I remembered what I had learned in yoga.

The Throat Mirrors the Birth Canal

Was I holding back somewhere? Was there something that I needed to say? I knew what it was right away and I called my husband over to me and told him how I felt. He was understanding and supportive. And what do you know, my labor kicked in a little while later.

Is there anything that you need to say but are holding back? As you explore this idea, consider if it's something you need to say aloud or just to yourself. And as you find your way through, know that the way you communicate matters just as much as your decision to do so. Be loving, and clear.

MANTRA: *I speak my truth compassionately.*

Rhythm, Ritual, and Relaxation

I attended a birth with a woman, bringing her third son into the world, but this would be the first time she would experience birth without medication. She was surprised by the sensations and at first looked outside herself to cope. She looked to her partner, she looked to the nurses, she looked at me. I looked right back at her and told her she's doing great. I grabbed her hand and said, "You can do this". I asked her husband to get a wet cloth for her neck while I provided counter-pressure on her back. I invited her between contractions to rest. And then when she felt the next one coming she looked at me, I reminded her, "You're doing great. Breathe."

Eventually she found her groove, as all women do...

Eventually she found her groove, as women tend to do. She found her rhythm, her ritual, and her way of relaxation. When a contraction would come she would begin her rhythm: swaying and moaning. Her ritual would be that she would grab my hand in one hand and her partner's in the other. She'd close her eyes and let her head hang, softening her shoulders and neck. When the contraction ended, she'd sit on a birthing ball, resting her head on the side of the bed. Through her rhythm, ritual, and relaxation she found her groove, and delivered her beautiful baby boy into her arms.

MANTRA: *I am one with the rhythm of the universe.*

Making Space

Clearing space in your mind is a goal of a Yoga practice. As time goes on, the beautiful spacious inner room of our minds becomes cluttered with the furniture of our experience (Eckhart Tolle). Experience is important and memories priceless, but in order to stay in the moment, and fully connect to our babies, we need to start letting go of the "stuff" that has piled up in our rooms.

Some examples I can think of for myself, are my opinion of myself as a mother. I have all this stuff built up in my mind, that's been building since childhood I imagine, of what a mother should be, and what kind of a mother I will be. Considering this is not a bad thing, and it's totally normal. However, it can become a problem when it gets in the way of our ability to enjoy where we're at right this very moment.

> *Don't judge it, just notice that it's there*

So as you go through your days, pregnant or not, notice the furniture in the room of your mind. Don't judge it, just notice that it's there. And from that awareness you can begin to make room.

Some of the best tools I've found to make room in the mind are breath utilization (see Chapter 8) and mantra.

MANTRA: *I am present in this moment.*

Ten

Foods for Your Body and Baby

*Please consult with your doctor before adding anything new in to your diet.

1st Trimester
Eat what you can when you can
Reduce processed foods
Reduce dairy if it is an issue for you
Add a Prenatal Multivitamin
Drink Fennel Tea for nausea
Balance beneficial gut bacteria with soup broths and quality Probiotics

2nd Trimester
Continue 1st Trimester Plan
Eat frequent small meals, let the largest meal be lunch
Increase cooked vegetables (including cooked greens)
Increase healthy oils like coconut, avocado, and olive oils

3rd Trimester
Continue 2nd Trimester Diet
Switch Fennel Tea for Red Raspberry Leaf Tea at 32 weeks (to tone uterus)

The following snack recipes can be enjoyed in between meals or with other foods.

* * *

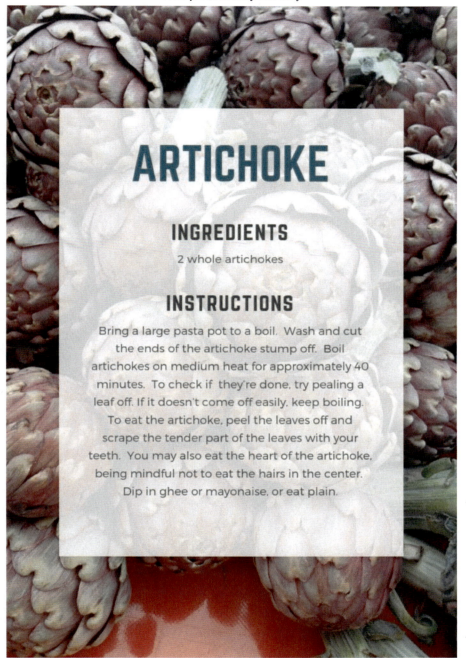

ARTICHOKE

INGREDIENTS

2 whole artichokes

INSTRUCTIONS

Bring a large pasta pot to a boil. Wash and cut the ends of the artichoke stump off. Boil artichokes on medium heat for approximately 40 minutes. To check if they're done, try pealing a leaf off. If it doesn't come off easily, keep boiling. To eat the artichoke, peel the leaves off and scrape the tender part of the leaves with your teeth. You may also eat the heart of the artichoke, being mindful not to eat the hairs in the center. Dip in ghee or mayonaise, or eat plain.

PICKLED GINGER CARROTS

INGREDIENTS

4 cups carrot sticks
1 tbsp freshly grated ginger
2 tbsp sea salt

INSTRUCTIONS

Mix ingredients in a metal bowl. Pound with a meat hammer to release juices. Place in a clean mason jar, and press down firmly until the juices cover the carrots. If they do not, add water until all the carrots are covered by 1 inch of liquid. Cover and keep at room temperature for 3 days. Place in the refrigerator to store.

SWEET POTATO FRIES

INGREDIENTS

1 Sweet Potato
1 tablespoon coconut oil
1/8 teaspoon tumeric
1/2 teaspoon ginger
1/8 teaspoon cinnamon
2 teaspoon cornstarch
1 tablespoon sea salt

INSTRUCTIONS

Clean the sweet potato and cut into ¼ inch sticks. Soak in water for 1 hour.
Preheat oven to 425. In a bowl, mix coconut oil and spices. In a separate bowl, mix sweet potato with cornstarch. Add the oil to the sweet potato and mix. Place the fries on a baking sheet keeping them spread evenly so they don't touch. Bake for about 25 minutes, flipping the sweet potatoes halfway through.

This recipe is adapted from Ayurveda Cooking for Beginners by Laura Plumb

PART III

Spirit Initiation

"We have not even to risk the adventure alone, for the heroes of all time have gone before us; the labyrinth is thoroughly known; we have only to follow the thread of the hero-path. And where we had thought to find an abomination, we shall find a God; where we had thought to slay another, we shall slay ourselves; where we had thought to travel outward, we shall come to the center of our own existence; where we had thought to be alone, we shall be with all the world."- Joseph Campbell.

Eleven

Stages of Receiving Spirit, the Hero's Journey

Becoming a mother is a call to adventure like none other. The *Spiritual Bootcamp* you have been experiencing is preparing you for your *Spirit Initiation*. *Spirit Initiation* is the moment, or collection of moments, where your skills that you have learned through pregnancy and life are utilized to take you from your ordinary world into a world where you become a hero. You'll use skills like trusting, letting go, being strong, breathing, using your voice, and staying present to help you cross the threshold from pregnancy and in to motherhood, embarking on a Hero's Journey.

The Hero's Journey taught by Joseph Campbell, in his comparative mythology texts, *The Hero With A Thousand Faces*, and *The Power of Myth*, is a metaphor for the deep inner journey of transformation and growth. The Journey transcends time and place, revealing a path on a journey we all share. You'll go from the "Ordinary World" and through a "Special World" until you ultimately return to the "Ordinary World" a changed person.

The deep inner transformation that a woman goes through during pregnancy, birth, and postpartum, is the Hero's Journey. Pam England teaches about this in her books *Birthing From Within* and *Ancient Maps for Modern Birth.* Each woman's birth is different, her strength will be tested in different ways (some physically, other's emotionally or spiritually). The birth story from one woman to the next will not the same, but the themes will be. Whether the birth is a Cesarean Birth, or even an adoption, the themes of going in to the unknown, being challenged, being triumphant, and then uncovering deep wisdom, all are found within the birth journey.

Stages of Receiving Spirit, the Hero's Journey

SPIRIT INITIATION

THE HERO'S JOURNEY

THE CALL TO ADVENTURE
The expecting mother is called from her ordinary life by contractions or water breaking. She doubts that it's happening.

TRANSFORM
In fear and bravery, you discover who you are, and use this powerful inner strength to bring baby into the world.

THE ORDEAL
She calls her partner/doctor/midwife/doula and enters her birth space. She is both brave and afraid.

THE HERO'S RETURN
You and your baby eat, rest, and get clean. You return home a new person.

- ORDINARY LIFE
- LOVE & WISDOM
- GROWTH
- HOMEWARD
- HOLDING BABY
- DELIVERY
- CONTRACTIONS START
- DOUBT
- CALL THE DR.
- ENTER BIRTH ROOM
- SENSATIONS OF BIRTH
- BABY APPROACHES

77

An Example of Birth As the Hero's Journey

{Ordinary World}

Ordinary World- A pregnant woman, 39 weeks along, moves differently now. She knows it could be any day that baby will come. There's an excitement and anticipation, but there's still grocery shopping to do, e-mails to check, and no baby snuggled up next to her yet. She's finishing putting the last few diapers in the diaper drawer, wondering if she has placed the mobile in the right spot.

Her Call to Adventure- The first contractions start.

Refuses the Call- She notices them and wonders if this is it or not. She decides its Braxton Hicks contractions and continues on her with her day. Now the contractions are regular and intensifying.

Calling the Mentor- She calls her partner, her doula, and her midwife. The doula and the partner arrive at the house and then the midwife.

Crossing the Threshold- The partner starts filling up the birthing tub as she watches in surprise that this is all happening. The doula massages her feet as the midwife checks the baby's heartbeat. Everything is normal and different all at once.

{Special World}

Being Tested- She sways through waves of confidence and fear. Her calm and strength are being tested.

Approaching the Inmost Cave- She dives into the strength of who she is as she enters the unknown. How long will this last? Will she be able to give birth vaginally? Is she okay? Is the baby okay? She has people around her that support her, but she knows it's up to her to do the work.

Ordeal- Her contractions strengthen and lengthen. Baby engages in the birth canal and eventually down to the vaginal opening. She battles her doubts and sensations. She uses her mantra and breath. *

Reward- Baby arrives into this world. 9 months of waiting is rewarded, and there is relief from the sensations of childbirth. She finds a sense of empowerment and a feeling of being loved.

{Return to Ordinary World}

The Road Back- She showers, eats, and revels in her baby. She slowly reemerges in the ordinary world, but the sense of trepidation about being a good mother lingers. Can she care for a newborn? Is she good enough?

Resurrection- She is deeply exhausted and a little uncertain about herself as the mother of an infant. But she continues bringing baby to her breast when he cries, changing his wet diapers, going to her appointments, and resting when baby rests. Ultimately she succeeds and emerges cleansed and reborn. She enjoys her first 6 weeks of motherhood by bonding with her baby, and letting people care for her.

Return with the Elixir- She has returned to the ordinary world a changed woman. She has learned many things, faced many challenges, and has grown as a person. She brings a new perspective for everyone to consider. She has let go of her self-doubt, reminding other people to trust themselves as well.

*Even an unexpected turn of events is a Hero's Journey- a hero is not in control, a hero is just willing to adapt and move forward. Your birth may happen differently than from what you expected- the Hero does not know what is before her, only that she must face it.

Twelve

Stages of Labor

Here is a map of the general stages of labor. It is helpful to familiarize yourself with these stages so that you can monitor yourself in every detail, but so that you have a broader knowledge that as labor progresses, your work and your sensations will adjust. There are many books about birth that go into more detail on the stages of labor and birth. This explanation is an overview to help you become comfortable with the stages of labor. The stages of labor are also taught as a part of most birth preparation classes.

The First Stage

Early Labor: This is the longest phase and typically lasts around half of the time most women are in labor. You will start to have contractions and they will become regular in occurrence. During this phase you will be able to do normal activities. Try to keep busy and distract yourself. Some women use this time to bake cookies for the staff that will be at the birth. Others fold baby clothes. You can save one of your easy tasks on your to-do list for this time. I've had women come to my Prenatal Yoga classes during early labor. If you can rest, rest; You're about to run a marathon.

- The cervix dilates between 0 and 4 cm.
- Contractions are distant, 10 to 20 minutes apart.

- Contractions are short only lasting 30 to 60 seconds long.
- Lasts 8 to 20 hours.

Active Labor: In this phase contractions become regular and more frequent. You will start the breathing techniques you have learned. This is also when you can go to your hospital or birth center (Especially, if you plan to get an epidural). Your body may slow contractions as you move from your home to your birth center/hospital. It takes some time and focus to get back in the groove.
- Dilation from 4 to 7 cm
- Contractions are closer together, 3 to 5 minutes apart
- Contractions are lasting about 60 seconds
- Can last 5-20 hours

Transition: This transition point is the hardest point before the birth of your baby. Thankfully, it is the shortest stage, lasting approx. 10 to 30 min (and it feels much shorter when you're going through it). The body is moving baby down and the pressure on the cervix invites it to open that final bit so that baby can move easily into the birth canal.
- Dilation 7 to 10 cm
- Contractions are close together, 1 to 3 minutes apart
- Contraction are lasting 90 seconds and are on/off/on/off
- Hormones may induce nausea and vomiting in some women
- Legs may tremble
- Hot or cold flushes
- Max time is 30 min

The Second Stage

This stage begins when the cervix is fully dilated, and ends when the baby is born. Your body will feel the urge to push the baby out. It will feel better to push than to stop yourself from pushing. This is when 'crowning' takes place. If you are having an un-medicated birth, you will feel your vaginal opening stretch. You'll move slowly to allow your body to do what it knows how to do. The techniques you used to practice focusing and relaxing will be very useful here. You can do anything one breath at a time. For women choosing an epidural, the doctor can direct your pushing, but many women are instead opting for *delayed pushing*, allowing the body to move the baby down on its own.

The Third Stage

This stage usually takes place between five minutes to 1 hour after birth. You will deliver the placenta and membranes that helped nourish your baby. For most women, baby is skin-to-skin on the mothers belly or chest during this final phase of birth.

Post-Partum: The post partum period can be defined as anywhere from 6 weeks to 3 years, depending on who you ask. The first 6weeks are considered the 4th trimester, or the sacred window. This is a time to stay in your bed, resting, eating warm foods, loving your baby, and staying warm. Leave the vacuum in the broom closet for those 6 weeks, it'll still be there when you've healed. Touch and ceremony are a great way to nourish yourself as you move through the post partum period.

Thirteen

Re-Birth in Postpartum

After giving birth, you enter the postpartum period. The first 6 weeks postpartum are considered the sacred window. It is a time for you and baby to bond, to snuggle, smell one another, and stay cozy. Emotions will fluctuate, as will your energy level. This sacred period for you and your baby can form a sort of cocoon for you and your baby to snuggle in to before re-emerging into the world. There are no rules, let yourself be free to explore your baby and yourself. This period of bonding between you and baby goes quick and yet some moments feel like years. So staying in the moment is important for your mind and body to adjust to this new life, and for baby to adjust to this new world. Notice the sounds your baby makes, the warm of baby's hands, the smell of baby's head, the feel of your own voice as you whisper, "I love you".

The following suggestions offer a couple of ways to help you and your baby make the most of this special time, marking the postpartum period as sacred. When we take the time to make moments in our lives sacred, we are able to slow down and let go of society's expectations of us, and we are able to fully be human. Maybe your religion or culture already has a way to help you through this sacred threshold. But most people in the West do not have this kind of ceremony passed down.

As you read through this section or explore other ideas online, decide what works for you. Here's a sample ceremony to consider.

SEALING CEREMONY

The sealing ceremony is an invitation to bring the birth process to a close. Birth is about being open, so we can balance this extreme experience by psychologically and physically closing the body, and integrating the birth experience. It can be done any time during the first 40 days post-partum.

If you have a moment or moments in your birth that are hard to move through physically or emotionally, it can be helpful to do some birth story sharing with a professional.

Ceremonial Bath

Have a close female friend or family run a bath for you with milk and honey added. Bring candles and any tokens or symbols that make you feel connected to birth and motherhood (pregnant photos, intergenerational photos, your hospital bracelet, a stone that is symbolic, a symbol of your faith etc.). Put on the music you listened to your during prenatal Yoga practice. Let your partner or other important people in your life bring you something sweet to drink. Review your birth in your mind, how your baby came into this world, and how you birthed him/her into it. Then use the glass to pour warm water over each part of your body that supported you in birth, offering gratitude to your body.

Tucking In

After your bath, invite your people to tuck you in with your baby. Place blankets and warm compresses (lightly warmed rice packs) over your bodies. Just as baby wants to be warm and held, your body will also benefit from feeling warm and held as you yourself are being born as the mother of this child.

It takes a couple of days for a baby to be born, it takes 6 weeks for a mother to be born. Especially the first time a woman becomes a mom, it takes her time to adjust to being responsible for an infant. But even with the second baby, or following babies, it is an adjustment to being the mother of this child. It takes time to learn which cries indicate stomach pain, hunger, or tiredness. It takes time to see yourself as a whole person and not just the caretaker of your baby. It takes time to find your rhythm, ritual, and relaxation in motherhood just as you do during birth. It also takes time for the body to close back up.

Foods for Postpartum

Cooked vegetables, congee, and warm foods all promote healing. If you can make food in advance and freeze it, that will help take some of the pressure off you during the post-partum period. If you notice people are offering to help you, ask them to make you some warm food to bring over during the first 6 weeks. You can even ask that they leave it on the doorstep as you might be sleeping.

Mantras for Post Partum

Use kind inner language as you navigate this new, beautiful, and challenging period. Use supportive and loving words. Try these mantras.

I am good enough.
I am capable.
I am breathing through this.
I am loving through this.
I am.

And sometimes the mantras for Post-Partum are: Please. Help. And, Thank You.

PART IV

Final Notes

The end of our exploring will be to arrive where we started and know the place for the first time- TS Eliot

Fourteen

Conclusion

Pregnancy is nature's way of preparing you for motherhood. It is Spiritual Bootcamp, training you for the initiation of birth, and the immense blessings of being Mother.

Our culture does not often support women in the deep spiritual work of pregnancy, birth, and motherhood. Find your tribe, and use this book as a resource to help you on your way.

Use the tools of Yoga in this book on a daily basis to help you on your Hero's Journey. Practice, even if it's for just a moment, and over time, you will have laid new neural pathways, making it easier to access these skills during your labor, and in motherhood. Find opportunities to practice the mental techniques as much as the physical ones. You can practice in the way you communicate with the people you love, in the way you focus your mind while you're waiting in line at the store, and even when you're having moments of discomfort in your body. Let go of the inner critic and replace those thoughts with the mantras in this book. You're exactly where you're meant to be, doing exactly what you need to do in this moment.

Namaste, the light of the universe that shines within me recognizes the light of the universe that shines within you and your baby, and it bows, thanking you. May this light inhabit our words, our thoughts, the space around us, bringing more peace and joy to the world.

Fifteen

About Lexi Meyerowitz

"A woman is like a teabag; you never know how strong it is until it's in hot water"
   -Eleanor Roosevelt

Hi, I'm Lexi Meyerowitz. I'm a San Diego prenatal yoga teacher and birth doula with two young daughters. I gave birth to Sophia Marley in 2012 and Hana Mei in 2015. The experiences of pregnancy, birth, and motherhood had parallel themes and life-lessons for me and it made me wonder if it's the universe's way of preparing us for the next stage.

   I have come to believe that this is so: pregnancy prepares us for birth, birth prepares us for motherhood, infants prepare us for toddlers, and so-on. That doesn't mean the transitions are easy, it just means we're supported on this epic Hero's Journey.

   In pregnancy I had to shield myself from other peoples' opinions. Strangers would tell me what to eat and how to exercise, completely unsolicited for this advise. I even had to shield myself from comments while I was in labor in the hospital elevator! Can you believe it?

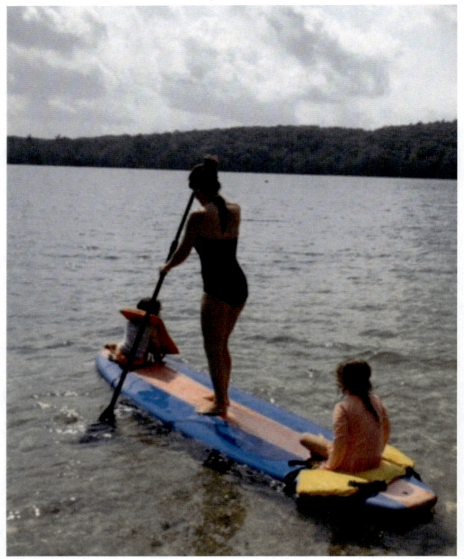

Stand Up Paddle Boarding with Sophia and Hana in CT.

In motherhood, I have had to respectfully ignore some peoples' advice, focusing instead on my own parental instincts (which are often quite spot-on). This theme of trusting intuition is one that comes up a lot in my life, and in particular in my journey into motherhood. It's the

Universe's way of reminding me to believe in myself.

I trusted my intuition to write *Spirit Birth*. Many Spirit Signals guided me to embark on the long process of learning about pregnancy and birth, writing, and releasing this book. And the compelling, intuitive, gut instinct to share this form of birth wisdom with other women drove this project forward. I have come to know that each woman has her own instincts and experiences to draw from, and it is part of my life's work to help women re-learn about, and *trust*, their intuition.

I have carried this intention into my parenting style. I believe that children are much closer and connected to universal energy than adults. And my goal with my own daughters, and the kids I work with at Hebrew school, is to trust in each child's own individual "Genius," and to create opportunities for them to explore and grow (see Reference-Rick Ackerly). This way, the children will learn to trust in their own intuition eventually.

Self-confidence and faith were other themes that arose frequently during pregnancy, birth, and the beginnings of motherhood for me. Self-confidence and intuition were related, because as I learned to follow my gut, I learned I could rely on myself. After each birth experience I felt invigorated by my own strength and courage, increasing my self-confidence.

But I think more than anything, it has been faith that carried me through the most challenging moments in pregnancy, birth, motherhood and life. When things don't seem to be going as I think they should, I pray to trust in the Universe. Now my trust in the Universe has waxed and waned, but faith was always present for me. I either had faith in a higher power, or faith in my family, or even my doctors, my husband, and my self.

Faith, self-confidence, and intuition helped me through my most difficult moments, and I feel like all of my experiences in birth and motherhood prepared me to deal with these unexpected crises.

First was Post-Partum Depression after my second birth. I felt increasingly isolated, and incapable, and until I asked for help so I could take a nap or go for a Yoga class, I thought I'd just have to make it work on my own. I believed in myself, but my intuition was telling me I needed help. I had faith in the process of counseling, so I found a specialist and began the work of taking better care of myself. I recall feeling like therapy was as relaxing as a day at the spa. It was like having a spiritual facial. And little did I know how important this safe space would become.

One night my husband wasn't feeling strange and went to bed early. I had the gut feeling that I should sit by the bed while he rested. My daughters were 3 and 1 and had just fallen asleep. I sat on the foot of our bed with my laptop, consulting Doctor Google, when suddenly my husband's body began to stiffen and rock. He moaned like he was starring in Poltergeist. I had no idea what was going on, just that I needed to protect his head from hitting the corner of the nightstand. My heart was pounding, but I held steady. I had no choice.

The ambulance was on its way shortly after that, and so were my parents, who would stay with my daughters that lay blissfully asleep. My girls had no idea that their world had drifted into chaos.

My husband is fine now, but this was the beginning of 2 years of struggle. There was a lot of waiting, waiting for tests, waiting for results, waiting for the city bus. I remember meditating and doing yoga in the waiting room while he went for his MRI. I had something I could hold on to, and that was my connection to the Universe.

There was a lot of change. My husband couldn't work temporarily, and his driver's license was taken away. The stress was palpable. There were so many moments of self-doubt, fear, and losing faith. But I knew I couldn't give up, I had my two beautiful daughters that lit up my world and I practiced having faith, following my intuition, and building up my self confidence. Now my husband is healthy, and everyone is doing well, including me. Through difficulties, I have learned how truly strong I am; I have discovered that I am heroic, just like you.

I am deeply thankful to the Universe for guiding me to this place, and I have faith in the Universe to continue to guide me forward.

Sixteen

Resources

RESOURCES

Your own Intuition and Wisdom

Birthing From Within- Pam England

Ayurveda Cooking for Beginners- Laura Plumb
   Nourishing Traditions- Sally Fallon

Finding a Birth Doula: DONA.org
   Getting Baby Into Optimum Position: SpinningBabies.com

Finding a Post-Partum Doula: DONA.org
   Post-Partum Depression/Anxiety: PostPartumHealthAlliance.org
   Post-Partum Ayurvedic Eating: PostPartumAyurveda.com

Meeting Other Moms: MeetUp.com

The Genius in Every Child- Rick Ackerly
   Conscious Parenting- Shefali Tsabary

The Power of Now - Echkart Tolle

Made in the USA
Coppell, TX
08 October 2024